HARNESSING THE POWER OF VITAMIN E

Your Essential Health and Wellness Companion

Dr. Raymond F. Bernard

TABLE OF CONTENTS

CHAPTER 1

Introduction to Vitamin E

Vitamins are essential nutrients that our bodies require in small quantities to function properly. One of these vital vitamins is Vitamin E. In this chapter, we will delve into the world of Vitamin E, understanding what it is, its historical significance, and the different forms it exists in.

What is Vitamin E?

Vitamin E is a fat-soluble vitamin that plays a crucial role in maintaining good health. It's often referred to as a "family" of compounds, consisting of four tocopherols (alpha, beta, gamma, and delta) and four tocotrienols (alpha, beta, gamma, and delta), each with varying levels of biological activity. These compounds are collectively known as Vitamin E, and they share a common antioxidant function.

Historical Background and Discovery

The history of Vitamin E is a fascinating journey that spans over a century. Its discovery can be attributed to several researchers, with significant contributions made by Herbert Evans and Katherine Bishop in the early 20th century.

In 1922, researchers Herbert McLean Evans and Katharine Scott Bishop were conducting experiments on rats to study their reproduction. They noticed that rats on a diet deficient in certain nutrients were unable to reproduce. When these rats were fed wheat germ, they not only regained their reproductive abilities but also produced healthy offspring. This led Evans and Bishop to discover a substance in wheat germ that was essential for reproduction. They named it "Vitamin E."

The term "Vitamin E" has a fascinating history in itself. The "E" in Vitamin E was assigned because it was the fifth vitamin to be discovered after Vitamins A, B, C, and D. In fact, Vitamins B and C were already known, but they had multiple subtypes, so Vitamin E was named sequentially.

The Importance of Vitamin E

Now that we understand the historical background, let's delve into why Vitamin E is so crucial for our health.

1. **Antioxidant Properties:** One of the primary roles of Vitamin E is its function as an antioxidant. Antioxidants are substances that protect our cells from oxidative stress caused by free radicals. Free radicals are unstable molecules that can damage cells, proteins, and DNA, leading to various diseases and aging. Vitamin E's antioxidant properties

help neutralize these harmful free radicals, reducing the risk of chronic diseases and promoting overall health.

2. **Immune System Support:** Vitamin E is also known for its immune-boosting properties. It helps regulate the immune system's response, enabling it to defend the body against infections and diseases effectively.

3. **Skin Health:** Vitamin E is often used in skincare products due to its ability to promote skin health. It can

help protect the skin from the damaging effects of UV radiation and promote skin repair and regeneration.

4. **Cardiovascular Health:** Studies have suggested that Vitamin E may play a role in reducing the risk of heart diseases by preventing the oxidation of LDL (low-density lipoprotein) cholesterol, often referred to as "bad" cholesterol. Oxidized LDL can contribute to the development of atherosclerosis, which is a major risk factor for heart disease.

5. **Neurological Health:** Some research has also explored the potential benefits of Vitamin E in maintaining cognitive function and reducing the risk of neurodegenerative diseases like Alzheimer's.

6. **Eye Health:** Vitamin E, along with other antioxidants like Vitamin C and zinc, has been associated with reducing the risk of age-related macular degeneration (AMD), a leading cause of vision loss in older adults.

7. **Cancer Prevention:** While research in this area is ongoing, Vitamin E's antioxidant properties have raised interest in its potential role in reducing the risk of certain cancers.

As we can see, Vitamin E is not just one-dimensional but rather a multi-faceted nutrient that contributes to overall health and well-being. Its role in maintaining various bodily functions makes it an essential part of our diet.

Forms of Vitamin E

Before we conclude this chapter, it's essential to understand that Vitamin E comes in different forms, each with its unique properties. The two primary groups of Vitamin E compounds are tocopherols and tocotrienols. Within these groups, there are four subtypes: alpha, beta, gamma, and delta.

Tocopherols are the most common form of Vitamin E found in nature, and alpha-tocopherol is the most biologically active form. It's the one most often associated with the health benefits of Vitamin E. Tocotrienols, on the other hand, are less common but have gained attention for their potential health benefits, especially in relation to heart health and cancer prevention.

In this book, we will explore these different forms of Vitamin E and their respective roles in maintaining health and preventing diseases.

As we conclude this chapter, it's clear that Vitamin E is not just a single nutrient but a complex family of compounds with diverse functions and a rich history of discovery. It's a vitamin that has fascinated scientists, health enthusiasts, and researchers for decades, and it continues to reveal its importance in maintaining and promoting human health. In the following chapters, we will dive deeper into the functions, sources, absorption, and potential risks and benefits of Vitamin E, equipping you with the knowledge to make informed decisions about your dietary choices and overall health.

CHAPTER 2

Functions and Benefits of Vitamin E

In this chapter, we will delve into the fascinating world of Vitamin E's functions and the numerous benefits it offers to our health. Vitamin E is often celebrated for its role as an antioxidant, but its influence on our well-being extends far beyond that.

The Multifaceted Role of Vitamin E

At its core, Vitamin E is renowned for its antioxidant properties. Antioxidants are substances that counteract the damaging effects of oxidative stress caused by free radicals. This oxidative stress can lead to cell damage, inflammation, and a wide range of health issues. Vitamin E, with its potent antioxidant abilities, stands as a guardian against this cellular damage.

1. Antioxidant Defense

Vitamin E's primary function is to protect our cells and tissues from oxidative damage. This damage can occur due to a variety of factors, including exposure to environmental toxins, pollution, UV radiation, and even normal metabolic processes within our bodies. When free radicals roam unchecked, they can attack and damage cellular components like DNA, proteins, and lipids, contributing to aging and various diseases.

Vitamin E swoops in to the rescue by neutralizing these free radicals, rendering them harmless. It donates an electron to the unstable free radicals, stabilizing them and preventing them from causing further damage. This antioxidant action helps maintain the integrity of our cells and tissues, promoting overall health and longevity.

2. Immune System Support

A strong and well-functioning immune system is essential for protecting our bodies against infections and diseases. Vitamin E plays a role in bolstering our immune defenses. It helps regulate immune responses and enhances the production of immune cells, ensuring that our body is prepared to combat invading pathogens effectively.

3. Skin Health and Beauty

Beautiful, healthy skin is a desire shared by many. Vitamin E has gained popularity in the skincare industry for its skin-nourishing properties. Here's how it contributes to skin health and beauty:

- **UV Protection:** Vitamin E acts as a natural sunscreen by absorbing harmful UV radiation. While it should not replace traditional sunscreens, it can provide an additional layer of protection against the sun's damaging effects.

- **Moisturization:** Vitamin E is often used in moisturizers and creams due to its ability to lock in moisture. It helps maintain skin hydration, preventing dryness and flakiness.

- **Wound Healing:** Vitamin E supports the healing of wounds, cuts, and burns. It promotes tissue repair and regeneration, reducing the appearance of scars.

- **Anti-Aging:** As an antioxidant, Vitamin E combats the signs of aging by protecting skin cells from oxidative stress. This can help reduce the development of wrinkles and fine lines.

4. Cardiovascular Health

Heart disease is a leading cause of mortality worldwide. Vitamin E contributes to cardiovascular health in several ways:

- **Cholesterol Regulation:** Vitamin E helps prevent the oxidation of LDL cholesterol, often referred to as "bad" cholesterol. Oxidized LDL cholesterol can contribute to the buildup of plaques in arteries (atherosclerosis), increasing the risk of heart disease.

- **Blood Vessel Health:** Vitamin E supports the proper functioning of blood vessels, helping to maintain their flexibility and preventing blood clots.

- **Blood Pressure Regulation:** Some studies suggest that Vitamin E may help regulate blood pressure, which is another critical factor in heart health.

5. Neurological Health

The brain is an energy-intensive organ and is susceptible to oxidative damage. Vitamin E may play a role in preserving cognitive function and reducing the risk of neurodegenerative diseases like Alzheimer's.

6. Eye Health

Age-related macular degeneration (AMD) is a leading cause of vision loss in older adults. Vitamin E, along with other antioxidants like Vitamin C and zinc, has been associated with a reduced risk of AMD. It helps protect the retina from oxidative damage and supports overall eye health.

7. Cancer Prevention

While research in this area is ongoing, Vitamin E's antioxidant properties have piqued interest in its potential role in reducing the risk of certain cancers. It is believed that Vitamin E's ability to neutralize free radicals may help prevent DNA damage and the development of cancerous cells.

8. Reproductive Health

Vitamin E is also important for reproductive health. It plays a role in the production of healthy sperm and may contribute to fertility.

9. Chronic Disease Prevention

The overall impact of Vitamin E on health is extensive. Its antioxidant and anti-inflammatory properties make it a potential player in reducing the risk of various chronic diseases, including diabetes, rheumatoid arthritis, and chronic obstructive pulmonary disease (COPD).

10. Overall Well-Being

Beyond its specific health benefits, Vitamin E contributes to our overall sense of well-being. When our bodies are protected from oxidative stress and inflammation, we are more likely to feel energetic, vibrant, and free from chronic health issues. This sense of well-being extends to our mental health as well, as physical health and mental health are intricately connected.

In summary, Vitamin E is a versatile and multifunctional nutrient that touches virtually every aspect of our health. From its role as a potent antioxidant to its contributions to cardiovascular health, skin beauty, and immune support, Vitamin E is a true champion of well-being. It underscores the importance of maintaining a balanced and nutrient-rich diet to ensure that our bodies receive an adequate supply of this vital vitamin. In the following chapters, we will explore the sources of Vitamin E in our diet, how our bodies absorb and utilize it, and how to maintain a healthy balance to reap its full benefits.

CHAPTER 3

Food Sources of Vitamin E

In this chapter, we will embark on a journey through the diverse landscape of food sources rich in Vitamin E. Understanding where to find this essential nutrient is fundamental for maintaining a healthy diet and reaping the benefits of Vitamin E's multifaceted roles in our well-being.

Why Food Sources Matter

Vitamin E is a fat-soluble vitamin, which means it dissolves in fats and oils. This characteristic has significant implications for its dietary sources and absorption in the body. Let's explore why food sources matter when it comes to Vitamin E.

Natural vs. Synthetic Vitamin E

Before we dive into specific foods, it's important to distinguish between natural and synthetic forms of Vitamin E. Natural Vitamin E, often labeled as "d-alpha-tocopherol," is derived from plant sources and is considered to be more biologically active and beneficial than its synthetic counterpart, known as "dl-alpha-tocopherol." When possible, it's advisable to opt for natural sources of Vitamin E in your diet.

Diverse Food Sources of Vitamin E

Vitamin E can be found in a wide range of foods, both plant-based and animal-based. Here are some of the most prominent sources:

1. Nuts and Seeds

Nuts and seeds are nutritional powerhouses and among the best sources of Vitamin E. Almonds, sunflower seeds, hazelnuts, and pine nuts are particularly rich in this nutrient. Just a small handful of these nuts or a sprinkle of seeds on your salad can provide a significant portion of your daily Vitamin E needs.

2. Vegetable Oils

Many cooking oils are excellent sources of Vitamin E, especially when they are cold-pressed or unrefined. Sunflower oil, wheat germ oil, safflower oil, and olive oil are notable examples. Incorporating these oils into your cooking and salad dressings can contribute to your Vitamin E intake.

3. Leafy Greens

Dark, leafy greens are not only rich in vitamins and minerals but also contain Vitamin E. Spinach, Swiss chard, and collard greens are some examples. Including these greens in your salads or as side dishes can boost your Vitamin E intake along with other essential nutrients.

4. Fortified Foods

Some processed foods, such as breakfast cereals and fruit juices, are fortified with Vitamin E. While these can be convenient sources, it's important to be mindful of the overall nutritional content of such products, as they may also contain added sugars and preservatives.

5. Fruits

Certain fruits contain modest amounts of Vitamin E. Kiwi, mangoes, and blackberries are examples. While fruits may not be as rich in Vitamin E as nuts and seeds, they still make valuable contributions to your overall intake.

6. Avocado

Avocado is a unique fruit in that it is rich in healthy fats, particularly monounsaturated fats. This makes it not only a good source of Vitamin E but also a nutritious addition to salads and sandwiches.

7. Whole Grains

Whole grains like wheat germ, brown rice, and oatmeal contain Vitamin E, albeit in smaller quantities compared to nuts and seeds. Choosing whole grains over refined grains can enhance your Vitamin E intake while providing other health benefits.

8. Seafood

While plant-based sources dominate the list, some seafood options also contain Vitamin E. Trout, salmon, and shrimp, for instance, provide this nutrient. However, the levels of Vitamin E in seafood are generally lower than in plant-based sources.

9. Eggs

Eggs are another source of Vitamin E, primarily found in the yolk. Incorporating eggs into your diet can provide you with a range of essential nutrients, including Vitamin E.

10. Dairy Products

Dairy products like milk and yogurt contain small amounts of Vitamin E. While they may not be the richest sources, they still contribute to your overall intake, especially if you consume them regularly.

11. Vegetables

Various vegetables, such as asparagus and red bell peppers, contain Vitamin E in smaller amounts. While they may not be the primary sources, including a variety of vegetables in your meals ensures a diverse nutrient intake.

12. Meat

Meat, particularly liver, contains Vitamin E. However, it's important to note that the levels of Vitamin E in meat are relatively low compared to other sources. If you consume meat, it can still contribute to your overall intake, but it's not the most efficient source.

Balancing Your Diet for Vitamin E

Achieving an optimal intake of Vitamin E involves balancing your diet with a variety of these food sources. A diverse diet not only ensures you get an adequate amount of Vitamin E but also provides a spectrum of other essential nutrients that work synergistically for your health.

Keep in mind that Vitamin E is best absorbed when consumed with dietary fats. This is because it's a fat-soluble vitamin, meaning it requires fats for proper absorption in the digestive tract. So, drizzling some olive oil on your salad or consuming nuts alongside your vegetables can enhance Vitamin E absorption.

Daily Intake Recommendations

The recommended daily intake of Vitamin E varies by age, sex, and life stage. On average, adult men and women should aim for around 15 milligrams (or 22.4 IU) of Vitamin E per day. Pregnant and lactating women may need slightly more.

It's important not to exceed the recommended daily intake, as excessive Vitamin E intake can have adverse effects. It's generally considered safe to obtain Vitamin E from dietary sources, but high-dose supplements should be used under the guidance of a healthcare professional.

Conclusion

In this chapter, we've explored the diverse array of food sources that provide us with the essential nutrient, Vitamin E. From nuts and seeds to leafy greens and vegetable oils, there are numerous options to incorporate into your diet to ensure you meet your Vitamin E needs. Choosing natural sources and maintaining a balanced diet is key to reaping the full benefits of this crucial nutrient.

In the subsequent chapters, we will delve deeper into the absorption and bioavailability of

Vitamin E, explore the consequences of deficiency and excess intake, and provide guidance on maintaining a balanced and healthful approach to Vitamin E consumption. Understanding the sources of Vitamin E is just the beginning of harnessing its potential for enhancing your overall well-being.

CHAPTER 4

Absorption and Bioavailability of Vitamin E

In this chapter, we will unravel the intricate process of how our bodies absorb and utilize Vitamin E, shedding light on the factors that influence its bioavailability. Understanding this aspect is crucial to making informed dietary choices and ensuring that you receive the maximum benefits from this essential nutrient.

The Digestive Journey of Vitamin E

Vitamin E is a fat-soluble vitamin, which means it is soluble in fats and oils but not in water. This characteristic affects how it is digested, absorbed, and transported within our bodies.

1. Digestion

The journey of Vitamin E begins in the stomach, where it encounters gastric juices and digestive enzymes. Unlike water-soluble vitamins, Vitamin E doesn't dissolve in the watery environment of the stomach.

Instead, it remains associated with dietary fats in the form of lipid droplets.

The majority of Vitamin E digestion and absorption occur in the small intestine, specifically in the upper part known as the duodenum. Here, bile produced by the liver and stored in the gallbladder is released to help emulsify dietary fats, breaking them down into smaller droplets. This process is critical for Vitamin E absorption because it disperses the fat-soluble vitamin within the digestive contents, making it accessible to enzymes that can break it down further.

2. Absorption

The absorption of Vitamin E primarily occurs in the brush border of the small intestine, which is densely packed with finger-like structures called villi and microvilli. These structures increase the surface area available for nutrient absorption.

Vitamin E is absorbed through a passive diffusion process, meaning it moves from an area of higher concentration (the digestive contents) to an area of lower concentration (the absorptive cells in the small intestine) without the need for energy.

Once absorbed by the cells of the small intestine, Vitamin E is then incorporated into chylomicrons, which are large lipoprotein particles. These chylomicrons transport Vitamin E, along with other dietary fats and fat-soluble vitamins, through the lymphatic system and into the bloodstream. From there, it is distributed to various tissues and organs throughout the body.

3. Transport and Storage

In the bloodstream, Vitamin E is carried by lipoproteins, with a significant portion associated with low-density lipoproteins (LDL) and high-density lipoproteins (HDL). These lipoproteins act as carriers, ensuring that Vitamin E reaches its target tissues and cells.

Vitamin E is also stored in the body, mainly in the liver and adipose (fat) tissue. This storage serves as a reserve for times when dietary intake may be insufficient.

Factors Influencing Vitamin E Bioavailability

Now that we've explored the digestive journey of Vitamin E, it's crucial to understand the factors that can influence its bioavailability—how much of the vitamin your body can actually absorb and use.

1. Dietary Fat Content

Since Vitamin E is fat-soluble, the presence of dietary fats in your meal significantly enhances its absorption. Therefore, consuming foods rich in Vitamin E with a source of healthy fats, such as olive oil or nuts, can increase its bioavailability.

2. Absorption Competition

Vitamin E absorption can be influenced by other fat-soluble vitamins, particularly Vitamin A. Excessive intake of one fat-soluble vitamin can interfere with the absorption of another. Therefore, maintaining a balanced intake of these vitamins is essential.

3. Fiber Intake

A diet high in dietary fiber, such as whole grains and fruits and vegetables, can affect Vitamin E absorption. Fiber can reduce the transit time of nutrients through the digestive tract, potentially limiting the time available for the absorption of Vitamin E. However, this effect is generally considered minor compared to the positive impact of a high-fiber diet on overall health.

4. Health Conditions

Certain health conditions can impair the absorption of dietary fat, and by extension, the absorption of fat-soluble vitamins like Vitamin E. Conditions like celiac disease, cystic fibrosis, and some pancreatic disorders can hinder fat absorption and, consequently, Vitamin E absorption. Individuals with these conditions may require specialized medical guidance to ensure adequate nutrient intake.

5. Age and Genetics

As we age, our digestive system may become less efficient at absorbing nutrients, including Vitamin E. Additionally, genetic factors can play a role in how well our bodies absorb and utilize this vitamin. Some individuals may have genetic variations that affect their Vitamin E metabolism.

6. Supplements vs. Food Sources

Vitamin E supplements are available in various forms, including synthetic and natural versions. Natural forms, such as d-alpha-tocopherol, are believed to be more biologically active and have higher bioavailability compared to synthetic forms (dl-alpha-tocopherol). However, the absorption of Vitamin E from supplements can still vary depending on the form and the presence of other nutrients or compounds.

Vitamin E Supplements and Bioavailability

It's important to note that while Vitamin E supplements can be a convenient way to boost your intake, they should be used judiciously. Excessive supplementation of Vitamin E can lead to adverse effects, including potential interference with blood clotting, gastrointestinal issues, and other health concerns.

Moreover, taking very high doses of Vitamin E supplements may not provide additional health benefits and could potentially be harmful. Therefore, it's advisable to obtain most of your Vitamin E from natural food sources and consider supplementation only when recommended by a healthcare professional.

Conclusion

In this chapter, we've unraveled the fascinating journey of Vitamin E from digestion to absorption and transport within our bodies. Understanding these processes and the factors that influence Vitamin E's bioavailability is crucial for making informed dietary choices.

To maximize the bioavailability of Vitamin E:

1. Consume a balanced diet rich in natural food sources of Vitamin E, including nuts, seeds, vegetable oils, leafy greens, and whole grains.

2. Include dietary fats, such as olive oil, avocados, and nuts, when consuming Vitamin E-rich foods.

3. Be mindful of any health conditions or medications that may affect fat absorption and nutrient utilization.

4. Consider supplementation only under the guidance of a healthcare professional and avoid excessive doses.

In the following chapters, we will explore the potential consequences of Vitamin E deficiency and excess, as well as provide practical guidance on maintaining a balanced intake of this essential nutrient to support your overall health and well-being. Understanding the intricacies of Vitamin E absorption and bioavailability is a crucial step toward optimizing its benefits for your health.

CHAPTER 5

Vitamin E Deficiency and Excess

In this chapter, we will delve into the consequences of both Vitamin E deficiency and excess. While Vitamin E is crucial for our health, maintaining the right balance is key. An imbalance can lead to health issues, so understanding the potential risks associated with deficiency and excess is vital.

Vitamin E Deficiency

Vitamin E deficiency occurs when the body doesn't receive an adequate amount of this essential nutrient over an extended period. Such a deficiency can have various causes and can manifest in several ways.

Causes of Vitamin E Deficiency

1. **Dietary Insufficiency:** The most common cause of Vitamin E deficiency is an inadequate dietary intake. This can happen if a person's diet lacks sufficient sources of Vitamin E-rich foods like

nuts, seeds, vegetable oils, and leafy greens.

2. **Malabsorption Issues:** Certain medical conditions, such as celiac disease, cystic fibrosis, and cholestatic liver disease, can impair the body's ability to absorb dietary fats and, consequently, fat-soluble vitamins like Vitamin E.

3. **Premature Infants:** Premature infants are particularly vulnerable to Vitamin E deficiency because they may not have had enough time in the womb to accumulate

sufficient stores of the vitamin. This deficiency can lead to a condition called hemolytic anemia, where red blood cells break down faster than the body can replace them.

Symptoms of Vitamin E Deficiency

The symptoms of Vitamin E deficiency can vary in severity. Common signs and symptoms include:

1. **Muscle Weakness:** Vitamin E plays a role in muscle function, and

deficiency can lead to muscle weakness and coordination problems.

2. **Vision Problems:** Vitamin E deficiency can affect the nerves responsible for eye muscle control, leading to difficulty in moving the eyes and, in severe cases, vision loss.

3. **Neurological Issues:** Vitamin E deficiency can impact the nervous system, leading to problems like impaired reflexes, difficulty walking, and muscle tremors.

4. **Anemia:** In some cases, Vitamin E deficiency can contribute to a form of anemia known as hemolytic anemia, where red blood cells break down prematurely.

5. **Immune System Compromise:** Vitamin E is essential for a robust immune system. A deficiency may weaken the body's defenses against infections.

Preventing Vitamin E Deficiency

Preventing Vitamin E deficiency involves ensuring an adequate intake of this essential nutrient through your diet. Incorporating foods rich in Vitamin E, such as nuts, seeds, vegetable oils, and leafy greens, can help maintain healthy Vitamin E levels.

In cases where malabsorption issues are present, medical intervention and dietary adjustments may be necessary. Premature infants and individuals with certain medical conditions may require Vitamin E supplementation under the guidance of a healthcare professional.

Vitamin E Excess

While Vitamin E is essential for health, excessive intake can lead to adverse effects. Vitamin E excess is relatively rare, primarily resulting from high-dose supplementation. Here are the potential risks associated with excessive Vitamin E intake:

1. Hemorrhage Risk:

One of the most significant concerns with excessive Vitamin E intake is an increased risk of bleeding or hemorrhage. Vitamin

E has anticoagulant properties, meaning it can interfere with blood clotting. This may be problematic for individuals on anticoagulant medications or those with bleeding disorders.

2. Gastrointestinal Issues:

High doses of Vitamin E supplements can cause digestive problems, such as nausea, diarrhea, and stomach cramps. These symptoms are usually temporary but can be uncomfortable.

3. Interference with Other Nutrients:

Excessive Vitamin E intake can interfere with the absorption and utilization of other fat-soluble vitamins, particularly Vitamin K. Vitamin K is essential for blood clotting, so Vitamin E's interference can exacerbate the risk of bleeding issues.

4. Increased Risk of Chronic Diseases:

There is some concern that very high doses of Vitamin E supplements may not provide additional health benefits and could even be harmful. Studies have raised questions about the potential association between high-dose Vitamin E supplementation and an increased risk of chronic diseases, such as prostate cancer and cardiovascular disease. However, the evidence in this area is complex and not entirely clear-cut.

5. Osteoporosis Risk:

Excessive Vitamin E intake may affect bone health. Some research suggests that very high doses of Vitamin E supplements may contribute to decreased bone density, potentially increasing the risk of osteoporosis. However, more research is needed to fully understand this relationship.

Balancing Your Vitamin E Intake

Maintaining a balanced intake of Vitamin E is essential for reaping its benefits without the risks associated with deficiency or excess. Here are some practical tips for ensuring a balanced approach to Vitamin E intake:

1. Prioritize Natural Food Sources:

The best way to obtain Vitamin E is through a well-rounded diet that includes natural food sources. Incorporate foods like nuts, seeds, vegetable oils, leafy greens, and whole grains into your meals to ensure you receive a consistent and balanced supply of Vitamin E.

2. Avoid Excessive Supplementation:

If you choose to take Vitamin E supplements, do so under the guidance of a healthcare professional. Avoid high-dose supplements unless specifically recommended for a medical condition.

3. Be Mindful of Multivitamins:

Check the labels of multivitamin supplements to ensure they

contain reasonable doses of Vitamin E and other vitamins and minerals. Avoid multivitamins with excessive amounts of Vitamin E, especially if you already have a balanced diet.

4. Consider Individual Health Needs:

Individual health conditions, such as malabsorption issues or dietary restrictions, may require special attention to Vitamin E intake. If you have specific health concerns, consult with a healthcare provider or registered dietitian for personalized guidance.

Conclusion

In this chapter, we've explored the potential consequences of both Vitamin E deficiency and excess. Maintaining the right balance of this essential nutrient is key to supporting your overall health and well-being. Vitamin E deficiency can lead to a range of health issues, including muscle weakness, vision problems, and neurological symptoms, while Vitamin E excess can result in an increased risk of bleeding and interference with other nutrients.

To maintain a balanced approach to Vitamin E intake:

- Include natural food sources in your diet, such as nuts, seeds, vegetable oils, and leafy greens.

- Avoid excessive supplementation and consult with a healthcare professional if considering high-dose supplements.

- Be mindful of multivitamin supplements and choose those with reasonable Vitamin E levels.

- Consider individual health needs and seek guidance if you have specific medical conditions or dietary restrictions.

In the following chapters, we will continue to explore the different facets of Vitamin E, including its functions in health and disease, as well as practical recommendations for maintaining a balanced and healthful approach to Vitamin E consumption. Understanding the potential risks and benefits of Vitamin E is essential for optimizing your well-being.

CHAPTER 6

Vitamin E Supplements

In this chapter, we will dive into the world of Vitamin E supplements. While obtaining Vitamin E from natural food sources is ideal, supplements can be a convenient way to ensure you meet your daily requirements. However, it's crucial to navigate the realm of supplements with knowledge and caution to maximize their benefits and avoid potential risks.

Understanding Vitamin E Supplements

Vitamin E supplements are readily available in various forms, including capsules, softgels, and liquid drops. These supplements typically contain synthetic forms of Vitamin E, such as dl-alpha-tocopherol, or natural forms, such as d-alpha-tocopherol. Understanding the differences between these forms is important, as they can impact their effectiveness in the body.

- **Natural vs. Synthetic Vitamin E:** Natural forms of Vitamin E, designated with a "d" prefix (e.g., d-alpha-tocopherol), are believed to be more biologically active and beneficial compared to synthetic forms, designated with a "dl" prefix (e.g., dl-alpha-tocopherol). The body may preferentially utilize natural Vitamin E. When choosing a supplement, it's generally recommended to opt for natural forms.

Vitamin E Supplement Benefits

Supplements can provide several benefits when used judiciously and under the guidance of a healthcare professional:

1. Meeting Dietary Needs:

Vitamin E supplements can help fill nutritional gaps in your diet, ensuring that you meet your daily requirements. This is particularly useful if you have dietary restrictions, malabsorption issues, or allergies that limit your intake of Vitamin E-rich foods.

2. Convenience:

Supplements offer a convenient way to obtain Vitamin E, especially for individuals with busy lifestyles or those who find it challenging to incorporate Vitamin E-rich foods into their daily meals.

3. Targeted Health Support:

In some cases, healthcare providers may recommend Vitamin E supplements for specific health conditions. For instance, Vitamin E supplements may be prescribed for individuals with Vitamin E deficiency, malabsorption disorders, or certain medical conditions that increase the body's Vitamin E requirements.

4. Skin Health:

Some people use Vitamin E supplements for their potential benefits for skin health. Vitamin E is known for its moisturizing and antioxidant properties, which may help with skin conditions and maintaining a youthful appearance.

5. Antioxidant Support:

Supplements can provide an extra boost of antioxidants, which can be particularly beneficial in situations of increased oxidative stress, such as recovery from illness or surgery.

Vitamin E Supplement Considerations

While Vitamin E supplements offer advantages, they should be used thoughtfully and within recommended guidelines. Here are some considerations when incorporating Vitamin E supplements into your routine:

1. Dietary Sources First:

Whenever possible, prioritize obtaining Vitamin E from natural food sources. A well-balanced diet provides a spectrum of nutrients and benefits that supplements cannot replicate. Supplements should complement, not replace, a healthy diet.

2. Recommended Dosages:

The recommended dietary allowance (RDA) for Vitamin E varies by age and sex but is generally around 15 milligrams (or 22.4 IU) per day for adults. Excessive supplementation can lead to potential risks, so it's essential to stay within recommended dosages.

3. Healthcare Professional Guidance:

Consult with a healthcare provider or registered dietitian before starting any Vitamin E supplement regimen, especially if you have underlying health conditions, are taking medications, or are pregnant or breastfeeding. They can provide personalized recommendations based on your specific needs.

4. Monitoring for Interactions:

Vitamin E supplements can interact with certain medications, such as blood thinners. It's essential to inform your healthcare provider about all supplements and medications you are taking to prevent potential interactions and adverse effects.

5. Quality Matters:

Choose reputable brands and products when selecting Vitamin E supplements. Look for supplements that clearly specify the form of Vitamin E (e.g., d-alpha-tocopherol) and avoid those with excessive dosages that far exceed the RDA.

6. Balanced Intake of Fat-Soluble Vitamins:

As a fat-soluble vitamin, Vitamin E interacts with other fat-soluble vitamins, such as Vitamin A and

Vitamin K. Maintaining a balanced intake of these vitamins is crucial to prevent imbalances and potential health issues.

7. Consideration for Specific Health Conditions:

Individuals with certain medical conditions may require specialized guidance on Vitamin E supplementation. For example, individuals with specific forms of malabsorption disorders may need higher doses under medical supervision.

8. Avoid Mega-Dosing:

Taking very high doses of Vitamin E supplements, often referred to as "mega-dosing," is not recommended unless specifically advised by a healthcare professional for a particular medical condition. Excessive supplementation can lead to adverse effects.

9. Potential Risks of Excess:

While Vitamin E is an essential nutrient, excessive supplementation has been associated with potential risks, including an increased risk of bleeding due to its anticoagulant properties. High-dose supplementation should be done under medical supervision.

Conclusion

In this chapter, we've explored the world of Vitamin E supplements, their benefits, and considerations for their use. Vitamin E supplements can be a valuable addition to your nutrition regimen when used thoughtfully and under the guidance of a healthcare professional.

Remember that natural food sources should always be your first choice for obtaining Vitamin E and other essential nutrients.

Supplements should be considered when dietary limitations or specific health conditions warrant them. To ensure a balanced approach to Vitamin E intake:

- Prioritize natural food sources like nuts, seeds, vegetable oils, and leafy greens.
- Consult with a healthcare provider before starting Vitamin E supplements, especially if you have underlying health conditions or are taking medications.
- Choose high-quality supplements that clearly

specify the form of Vitamin E and stay within recommended dosages.

In the following chapters, we will continue our exploration of Vitamin E, including its roles in health and disease, practical dietary recommendations, and guidance on maintaining a balanced approach to Vitamin E consumption. Understanding the benefits and potential risks of Vitamin E supplements is essential for optimizing your overall well-being.

CHAPTER 7

Vitamin E in Health and Disease

In this chapter, we will explore the significant roles Vitamin E plays in maintaining health and its potential impact on various diseases. Vitamin E is more than just an antioxidant; it has a multifaceted influence on our well-being, affecting everything from our immune system to our cardiovascular health.

Vitamin E and Antioxidant Defense

At its core, Vitamin E is renowned for its role as an antioxidant. Antioxidants are substances that neutralize harmful free radicals in our bodies, protecting our cells and tissues from oxidative damage. This primary function forms the basis of Vitamin E's influence on health.

1. Cellular Protection

Free radicals are highly reactive molecules produced as natural byproducts of metabolism and from external sources like UV radiation and pollution. When left unchecked, they can cause oxidative stress, damaging cellular components like DNA, proteins, and lipids. Vitamin E swoops in as a guardian, donating electrons to stabilize these free radicals, preventing further damage to our cells.

By safeguarding the integrity of our cells, Vitamin E helps reduce the risk of various chronic diseases and supports overall well-being.

Vitamin E and Immune Health

A strong immune system is essential for defending our bodies against infections and diseases. Vitamin E contributes to immune function in several ways:

1. Immune Cell Function

Vitamin E supports the proper functioning of various immune cells, including T cells and B cells. These cells are responsible for identifying and neutralizing pathogens like bacteria and viruses.

2. Antibody Production

Vitamin E also plays a role in antibody production, enhancing the body's ability to recognize and respond to invaders.

3. Immune Regulation

Vitamin E helps regulate immune responses, preventing overactivity that can lead to chronic inflammation and autoimmune diseases.

Vitamin E and Skin Health

Our skin is our body's largest organ, and its health is a reflection of our overall well-being. Vitamin E is celebrated in the skincare industry for its contributions to skin health:

1. UV Protection

Vitamin E acts as a natural sunscreen, absorbing harmful UV radiation. While it should not replace traditional sunscreens, it provides an extra layer of protection against the sun's damaging effects.

2. Moisturization

Vitamin E is often included in moisturizers and creams due to its ability to lock in moisture. It helps maintain skin hydration, preventing dryness and flakiness.

3. Wound Healing

Vitamin E supports the healing of wounds, cuts, and burns. It promotes tissue repair and regeneration, reducing the appearance of scars.

4. Anti-Aging

As an antioxidant, Vitamin E combats the signs of aging by protecting skin cells from oxidative stress. This can help reduce the development of wrinkles and fine lines.

Vitamin E and Cardiovascular Health

Heart disease is a leading cause of mortality worldwide, making cardiovascular health a paramount concern. Vitamin E contributes to cardiovascular well-being in several ways:

1. Cholesterol Regulation

Vitamin E helps prevent the oxidation of LDL cholesterol, often referred to as "bad" cholesterol. Oxidized LDL cholesterol can contribute to the buildup of plaques in arteries (atherosclerosis), increasing the risk of heart disease.

2. Blood Vessel Health

Vitamin E supports the proper functioning of blood vessels,

helping to maintain their flexibility and preventing blood clots.

3. Blood Pressure Regulation

Some studies suggest that Vitamin E may help regulate blood pressure, which is another critical factor in heart health.

Vitamin E and Neurological Health

The brain is an energy-intensive organ and is susceptible to oxidative damage. Vitamin E may play a role in preserving cognitive function and reducing the risk of neurodegenerative diseases like Alzheimer's.

Vitamin E and Eye Health

Age-related macular degeneration (AMD) is a leading cause of vision loss in older adults. Vitamin E, along with other antioxidants like Vitamin C and zinc, has been associated with a reduced risk of AMD. It helps protect the retina from oxidative damage and supports overall eye health.

Vitamin E and Cancer Prevention

Research in this area is ongoing, but Vitamin E's antioxidant properties have sparked interest in its potential role in reducing the risk of certain cancers. It is believed that Vitamin E's ability to neutralize free radicals may help prevent DNA damage and the development of cancerous cells.

Vitamin E and Reproductive Health

Vitamin E is also important for reproductive health. It plays a role in the production of healthy sperm and may contribute to fertility.

Vitamin E and Chronic Disease Prevention

The overall impact of Vitamin E on health is extensive. Its antioxidant and anti-inflammatory properties make it a potential player in reducing the risk of various chronic diseases, including diabetes, rheumatoid arthritis, and chronic obstructive pulmonary disease (COPD).

Vitamin E in Disease Management

In addition to its role in preventing diseases, Vitamin E can also be beneficial in managing certain health conditions:

1. Alzheimer's Disease

Some studies suggest that Vitamin E may slow the progression of Alzheimer's disease and improve cognitive function in individuals with this condition. However, more research is needed in this area.

2. Non-Alcoholic Fatty Liver Disease (NAFLD)

NAFLD is a condition characterized by the accumulation of fat in the liver. Vitamin E has been used in the management of NAFLD, as it may help reduce liver inflammation and oxidative stress.

3. Menstrual Pain (Dysmenorrhea)

Vitamin E supplements have been investigated for their potential to alleviate menstrual pain and discomfort, with some studies showing promising results.

4. Cataracts

Research suggests that Vitamin E may help reduce the risk of developing cataracts, a common eye condition characterized by clouding of the lens.

Conclusion

In this chapter, we've explored the significant roles Vitamin E plays in maintaining health and its potential impact on various diseases. Vitamin E's influence extends far beyond its antioxidant properties, touching virtually every aspect of our well-being, from our immune system and cardiovascular health to skin beauty and neurological function.

Understanding the multifaceted benefits of Vitamin E underscores the importance of maintaining a balanced and nutrient-rich diet to ensure that our bodies receive an adequate supply of this vital vitamin. In the following chapters, we will continue our exploration of Vitamin E, including practical dietary recommendations, guidance on Vitamin E supplementation, and strategies for maintaining a balanced approach to Vitamin E consumption. Embracing the full potential of Vitamin E can enhance your overall health and well-being, supporting a vibrant and fulfilling life.

CHAPTER 8

Practical Dietary Recommendations for Vitamin E

In this final chapter of our exploration of Vitamin E, we will provide practical dietary recommendations to help you incorporate this essential nutrient into your daily life effectively. A balanced diet rich in Vitamin E is key to reaping its numerous health benefits while avoiding the risks of deficiency or excess.

1. Diverse Food Sources

The first and foremost recommendation for obtaining Vitamin E is to diversify your food choices. Vitamin E is found in a wide range of foods, both plant-based and animal-based. Including a variety of these foods in your diet ensures that you receive a spectrum of nutrients, including Vitamin E.

Here are some Vitamin E-rich foods to consider:

- **Nuts and Seeds:** Almonds, sunflower seeds, hazelnuts, and pumpkin seeds are excellent sources of Vitamin E. Snack on a handful of these nuts or sprinkle seeds on your yogurt or salads.

- **Vegetable Oils:** Cooking with oils like sunflower oil, wheat germ oil, safflower oil, and olive oil can boost your Vitamin E intake. Use them in salad dressings and for sautéing vegetables.

- **Leafy Greens:** Incorporate dark, leafy greens like spinach, Swiss chard, and collard greens into your salads, stir-fries, and smoothies to increase your Vitamin E consumption.

- **Whole Grains:** Opt for whole grains like wheat germ, brown rice, and oatmeal over refined grains in your meals. These grains contain Vitamin E in addition to other essential nutrients.

- **Avocado:** Avocado is not only delicious but also a nutritious source of healthy fats and Vitamin E. Enjoy it in sandwiches, salads, or as a topping for toast.

- **Fruits:** While fruits generally contain smaller amounts of Vitamin E compared to nuts and seeds, they still make valuable contributions. Kiwi, mangoes, and blackberries are examples of fruits with modest Vitamin E content.

- **Eggs:** Eggs, particularly the yolk, contain Vitamin E. Include eggs in your diet for a range of essential nutrients, including protein and Vitamin E.

- **Seafood:** Some seafood options like trout, salmon, and shrimp provide Vitamin E, although in smaller quantities compared to plant-based sources.

- **Meat:** Meat, especially liver, contains Vitamin E, but it's generally not the most efficient source compared to plant-based options.

- **Dairy Products:** Milk and yogurt contain small amounts of Vitamin E. If you consume dairy, it can still contribute to your overall intake.

- **Vegetables:** Various vegetables, including asparagus and red bell peppers, contain Vitamin E in smaller amounts. A variety of vegetables in your meals ensures diverse nutrient intake.

2. Balanced Diet with Healthy Fats

Vitamin E is a fat-soluble vitamin, meaning it requires fats for proper absorption in the digestive tract. To enhance Vitamin E absorption, include healthy fats in your diet. Olive oil, avocados, nuts, and seeds are excellent sources of both healthy fats and Vitamin E. Consider drizzling olive oil on your salads or adding nuts and seeds to your meals to maximize absorption.

3. Cooking Techniques

Be mindful of your cooking techniques to retain Vitamin E in your foods. Steaming, sautéing, and roasting vegetables are better options than boiling, as Vitamin E can leach into the cooking water. When using oils for cooking, opt for low to medium heat to prevent excessive degradation of the vitamin.

4. Minimize Food Processing

Processed foods can lose significant amounts of Vitamin E during manufacturing. Whenever possible, choose whole, minimally processed foods over heavily processed options. For example, whole grains contain more Vitamin E than highly refined grains.

5. Dietary Supplements

While whole foods should be your primary source of nutrients, there are cases where dietary supplements may be appropriate:

- **Deficiency:** If you have a diagnosed Vitamin E deficiency, your healthcare provider may recommend supplements to restore your Vitamin E levels.

- **Medical Conditions:** Certain medical conditions, such as malabsorption disorders, may require supplementation under medical supervision.

- **Specific Dietary Restrictions:** Individuals with strict dietary restrictions, such as vegan diets, may consider supplements to ensure they meet their Vitamin E needs.

Always consult with a healthcare professional before starting any dietary supplement regimen. Excessive supplementation can have adverse effects, and it's important to determine the appropriate dosage based on your specific health needs.

6. Daily Intake Recommendations

The recommended daily intake of Vitamin E varies by age, sex, and life stage. On average, adult men and women should aim for around 15 milligrams (or 22.4 IU) of Vitamin E per day. Pregnant and lactating women may need slightly more.

7. Be Mindful of Interactions

Vitamin E can interact with certain medications and other nutrients. For example, it can interfere with blood thinners, increasing the risk of bleeding. Inform your healthcare provider about all supplements and medications you are taking to prevent potential interactions and adverse effects.

8. Individualized Approach

Individual health conditions, dietary preferences, and lifestyle factors can influence your Vitamin E needs. If you have specific health concerns, consult with a registered dietitian or healthcare provider for personalized guidance on Vitamin E intake.

9. Avoid Mega-Dosing

Taking very high doses of Vitamin E supplements, often referred to as "mega-dosing," is not recommended unless specifically advised by a healthcare professional for a particular medical condition. Excessive supplementation can lead to adverse effects, including an increased risk of bleeding due to Vitamin E's anticoagulant properties.

10. Balance with Other Nutrients

Vitamin E interacts with other fat-soluble vitamins, such as Vitamin A and Vitamin K. Maintaining a balanced intake of these vitamins is crucial to prevent imbalances and potential health issues. A well-rounded diet should provide this balance naturally.

Conclusion

In this final chapter, we've provided practical dietary recommendations for incorporating Vitamin E into your daily life effectively. Vitamin E is an essential nutrient with a wide range of health benefits, and a balanced diet rich in diverse food sources is the best way to ensure you receive its full advantages.

By diversifying your food choices, including healthy fats, and mindful cooking techniques, you can maximize your Vitamin E intake. While supplements may be necessary in certain situations, whole foods should be your primary source of this essential nutrient. Always consult with a healthcare professional for personalized guidance on Vitamin E intake, especially if you have specific health conditions or dietary restrictions.

Maintaining a balanced approach to Vitamin E consumption is essential for optimizing your overall health and well-being. Embracing the full potential of Vitamin E can support a vibrant and fulfilling life, keeping you in the best possible health for years to come.

CONCLUSION

In conclusion, Vitamin E is a versatile and essential nutrient that plays a crucial role in maintaining our health and well-being. Throughout this book, we've explored the various facets of Vitamin E, from its functions as an antioxidant and immune system supporter to its influence on cardiovascular health, skin beauty, and more.

Understanding the importance of Vitamin E in our diet is paramount. Incorporating diverse food sources, such as nuts, seeds, vegetable oils, leafy greens, and whole grains, is the foundation for ensuring an adequate intake of this vital vitamin. Balanced dietary choices, along with healthy fats and cooking techniques that preserve Vitamin E, contribute to its effective absorption and utilization in the body.

While whole foods should be the primary source of nutrients, there are situations where Vitamin E supplements may be necessary, such as in cases of deficiency or specific medical conditions. However, it's crucial to use supplements judiciously and under the guidance of a healthcare professional to avoid potential risks associated with excessive intake.

Maintaining a balanced approach to Vitamin E consumption involves being mindful of individual health needs, potential interactions with medications, and the importance of achieving a harmonious intake of other fat-soluble vitamins.

By embracing the full potential of Vitamin E through a well-rounded diet and informed supplementation when necessary, you can optimize your overall health and well-being. Vitamin E is a valuable ally in your quest for a vibrant and fulfilling life, supporting your body in staying healthy and resilient for years to come.

www.ingramcontent.com/pod-product-compliance
Lightning Source LLC
Chambersburg PA
CBHW050922260726
48660CB00001B/338